Meaningful Connections

Positive Ways to be Together
When a Loved One has Dementia

Other books by Nancy Kriseman

The Caring Spirit Approach to Eldercare: A Training Guide for Professionals and Families

The Mindful Caregiver: Finding Ease in the Caregiving Journey

Meaningful Connections

Positive Ways to be Together
When a Loved One has Dementia

Nancy L. Kriseman, LCSW

Published by Geriatric Consulting Services, Inc.

Library of Congress Control Number: 2017903191

Kriseman, Nancy, author.

   Meaningful Connections: Positive Ways To Be Together When A Loved One Has Dementia / by Nancy L Kriseman

   p. cm.

   "A practical guide on how to engage and create meaningful connections when caring for a loved one with dementia."

   1. Dementia--Care 2. Caregivers--Psychology. 3. Aging parents--Care. 4 Adult children of aging parents--Family relationships. 5.Self Care--Methods. 6. Alzheimer's Disease. I. Title

ISBN-13: 978-0998696201 (Paperbook)

ISBN-13: 978-0-998696218 (Electronic Book)

Printed in the United States of America

To all those who have dementia
and their care partners.
May you find meaningful connections
and positive ways to be together!

Contents

Acknowledgments

Every author knows that it takes a village to publish a book. And I have been extremely blessed with all the people who have supported me. My amazing friends and colleagues encouraged me, nourished my spirit and listened to endless updates about the book. They are too numerous to mention each by name, but they know who they are. I do, however, want to especially thank a few individuals.

First, I must acknowledge my partner, Cynthia Jorgensen, who I appreciate and treasure with all my heart. She gave endless hours of her time, providing thoughtful input, a critical eye and editorial suggestions to help make the book practical and easy to read. No words can adequately express my deep appreciation and gratitude.

I can't thank enough, my amazing graphic book designer, Ines Kuhn. Not only is she extremely creative and skillful at her craft, she has an incredibly generous and caring heart. Ines went above and beyond to make this book come alive! And did so with a loving spirit.

What can I say about my dear friend Isabel Chason, retired school teacher, and a care partner to her mother's sister. Isabel is such a generous and loving soul. When I shared my idea about this book, Isabel didn't hesitate to offer her time and talent. She helped create and design the Grab & Go Activity Boxes, and spent endless hours finding invaluable resources. Isabel is truly what I call a "caring spirit."

Thank you to my readers and reviewers: Jackie Pinkowitz, Chair of Dementia Action Alliance, (colleague and care partner for her mother and father-in-law); Dr. Hal Rogers, Director, Psychology Clinic, Georgia State University (colleague and a family care partner); Suzette Binford, Program Director for Early Stage Dementia, Georgia Alzheimer's Association; and Bonnie Cooper, a fellow social worker and my dearest friend. They gave of their time, reading through the book, offering excellent suggestions, and writing thoughtful reviews.

My copy editor and good friend, Vicki Clemmer, a retired journalist, graciously gave her time and talent to copy edit my book.

Last, but certainly not least, is Lou Brown Jewel, who cared for her first husband Worley, who had dementia and was a caregiver for her second husband as well. She has been a champion for caregivers all her life, donating her time and money to this cause. She is my "book angel."

Meaningful Connections: An Introduction

IF you are reading this book, then I suspect you have a loved one with dementia. Whether you are a family member, friend, neighbor or professional, this book is for you, the care partner – the preferred name for caregivers.

This book was inspired by my professional and personal experiences as a Geriatric Clinical Social Worker and as a daughter of mother with Alzheimer's. I have worked in the field of aging for more than 30 years, and specialize in working with families caring for someone with dementia. In addition, my mother was diagnosed with Alzheimer's at age 71 and lived with the disease for 17 years. As her dementia progressed, I quickly realized that spending time together without a specific plan was often unpleasant for us both. So, I sought out ways to have more meaningful connections with my mother. I realized I had to be *intentional* with my visits, and mindful of her strengths and abilities. Being intentional meant that I had to *plan my visits*. For example, my mother loved being outside, so I often would bring a picnic lunch to eat together in the garden, along with listening to her favorite music. Planning my visits helped me to focus on other ways to encourage more enjoyable and meaningful time together. I realized this would hold true for many of my clients as well. I want to share my ideas and tips, as well as the wonderful suggestions that care partners have taught me, so that you may learn from us all.

How this Book Can Help You

My hope is that this book will help you find new ways to spend time with your loved one when his or her dementia has progressed to a point where spending time together is challenging. In the early stages of cognitive impairment, engagement can mean adapting to the new normal. But when the disease progresses to a point where your loved one is requiring supervised care or needs to be in a residential community, new ways to engage may be required. As a spousal caregiver said, "we have to learn to love them where they are."

Each chapter offers ideas, examples and resources to make your time together truly matter! While this book is intended to be focused on helping care partners visit with a loved one in a residential community, much of what I offer also applies to people living at home. Note that throughout this book, I alternate between "he" and "she" to be gender neutral.

I encourage you to read whatever chapter might be the most helpful to you. Some people might want to read the book from beginning to end. Others may want to read the chapter most relevant to their concerns. Below are descriptions of the book's content.

Chapter 1: Understanding How Dementia Affects Engagement

This chapter describes how your loved one's abilities and capabilities can affect how you spend time together. The Dementia Abilities Continuum describes three stages of cognitive functioning and provides questions to help you assess your loved one's cognitive abilities. The continuum outlines how dementia can progress and what you might expect at each stage. It is also designed to help you determine the type of engagement and activities that are appropriate for your loved one.

Chapter 2: How to Visit with a Loved One who has Dementia

The goal of this chapter is feeling more ease when visiting your loved one. There are tips on making the most of your visits. I will provide some of the common questions from care partners, along with the answers. In addition, there is information about how to visit when there are special situations, such as when a loved is agitated, sleeping excessively or can't verbally communicate.

Chapter 3: Meaningful Engagement and Person-Centered Activities

Meaningful engagement and person-centered activities are two important concepts that can enhance your connections. These terms are explained, along with suggestions on how to best interact with people who have dementia. *Meaningful engagement* requires assessing your loved one's abilities and matching activities that maximize mutual enjoyment. *Person-centered activities* focus on choosing specific activities from your loved one's interests, past life experiences, career and hobbies. This chapter highlights how you and your loved one can benefit from this approach. Appendix A, includes examples of how to personalize your visits by creating simple 'Grab & Go Activity Boxes.'

Chapter 4: Creating Person-Centered Activities

This chapter builds upon the previous content and introduces practical tips about how to provide person-centered activities. A description of different categories of activities allows you to pick and choose which ones best match your loved one's interests and abilities. Each category is described, along with suggestions for engagement and supply items to help implement the activity. In addition, there are examples of how to adapt an activity to the changing cognitive abilities of your loved one.

Chapter 5: Recognizing Your Own Feelings

This chapter explores the different and sometimes complicated feelings that can arise from caring for someone who has dementia. There can be situations when meaningful engagement may be difficult. Being aware of the reasons you may feel certain ways, and how to handle these situations, is the focus of this chapter. Additionally, I touch on the difficult topic of estranged or abusive relationships.

Chapter 6: Finding Ease with Your Loved One at the End of Life

It is not easy to be with someone you love at the end of life. This chapter provides ideas about how to visit with your loved one during this extraordinarily special, but difficult time. There is also some information about hospice, which can be another way to support you and your loved one during this time.

Appendix A: Grab & Go Activity Boxes

Grab & Go Activity Boxes are theme related boxes that you create and bring when you visit with your loved one. You then use the items in the box to help stimulate memories and conversation. It can be fun to take turns picking out items and using them to engage your loved one. Included are pictures and descriptions of four different Grab & Go Activity Boxes, as well as suggestions for items and ways to enhance your time together.

Appendix B: Websites and Resources

This appendix offers some websites from which you can order activity supplies. Additionally, there are some suggestions to get you jump-started on expanding your thinking about other ways to engage with your loved one.

Chapter 1

Understanding How Dementia Affects Engagement

"We thrive when we
feel intimately connected
heart to heart and
soul to soul"

-Paula Reeves, Heart Sense

WHEN someone has dementia and it has progressed so that the person requires more care and supervision, it can be difficult to connect to him or her. Carrying on a conversation or enjoying passing the time together may be more challenging. Yet most care partners want to be able to spend meaningful time with their loved ones. With some knowledge and experience, you can connect in meaningful ways.

Thinking Differently About Those Living with Dementia

People living with dementia express the importance of being treated with respect and as a whole person, especially as their cognition declines. They don't want to be known as a "dementia victim," "patient," or "sufferer." They want the opportunity to experience living as fully as possible – even with their dementia. As dementia and cognitive impairment progresses, as it almost always does, it will be important to adjust your thinking about your loved one. Focusing on your loved one's *strengths* and *abilities* (vs. weaknesses and disabilities), allows you to support your loved one so that she can hold on to her personhood. This requires looking for opportunities for her to be successful. For example, you may no longer be able to hold conversations with her; however, she may enjoy you reading to her. Whether she remembers what is read to her is not as essential as her enjoying herself. So, it is important to find activities that match your loved one's abilities. Let me share a personal example.

My mother lived with Alzheimer's disease for 17 years, and throughout this journey, I wanted to find ways to stay positively connected to her. This meant paying close attention to her abilities and strengths. My mother enjoyed being outdoors, so we spent a lot of time going to parks, strolling on the beach, and exploring the gardens of her residential community. When she could no longer walk, and was in a wheel chair, I couldn't take her to the beach, but we could still take wheel chair strolls outside. I wanted to make sure I honored her love for the outdoors and continued to find ways to connect that were meaningful. At the end of my mother's life, when illness confined her to her room, I brought the outdoors in. I filled her room with plants and flowers, a small water fountain, and lavender and other flower scents.

Learning to Observe

It is essential for care partners to learn to be good observers and pay attention to their loved ones' physical, cognitive, and social well-being. The questions below can help you determine their abilities.

As you work through these questions, I suggest that you write down your answers. This will help you consider ways to tailor your visit and interactions. Be mindful that over time, your loved one's abilities and capabilities will change and so will your answers.

Physical Questions

What physical challenges does your loved one have that can impact her ability to participate in activities and engagement?

– Does she have trouble hearing? Hearing abilities can certainly influence how well she will understand the information shared.

– Is her eyesight impaired? If she has trouble seeing, she can become more easily frightened or fearful, especially by sudden movements.

– Does she have special dietary requirements, such as a soft diet? This might mean planning ahead for outings that include meals.

– Is she prone to wandering or pacing? If so she can be at risk for getting lost or hurt.

– Does she have balance issues? Lack of balance can increase her risk for falling.

– Is she incontinent of bowel or bladder? This can restrict where you are able to take her.

Cognitive Questions

There are many cognitive symptoms of dementia that can impact engagement.

- Does he have short-term memory issues such as forgetting appointments, forgetting what you just talked about, or asking the same questions over and over?

- Can he follow conversations or understand verbal information? Is he able to process the information?

- Does he exhibit long-term memory issues, such as not remembering his family members, being unable to share where he grew up, or forgetting what career he had?

- Does he remember to take his medications as prescribed? Is he able to manage having medicines refilled in a timely manner?

- How long is his attention span? Can he remember what he has just read? Can he watch a movie or program through its entirety? Does he become easily distracted?

- Does he exhibit confusion and disorientation such as not knowing where he is, thinking he is still working, or thinking it is nighttime when it is daytime?

- Does he have difficulty with verbal expression? Does he mix up words in sentences, call objects by the wrong names, or struggle with expressing himself?

- Does he have some challenges with what are labeled as executive functions? For example, does he have difficulty with judgement and reasoning? Does he make impulsive decisions? Is he able to assess his safety?

- Does he have trouble performing familiar or routine tasks, such as keeping track of finances, paying bills, working the stove or microwave, or using the TV remote?

Social Questions

Researchers have demonstrated the importance of social interaction and engagement. Finding ways to keep your loved one engaged and involved in activities can have numerous positive effects. Here are some questions for your consideration about your loved one's social interactions.

- Is she still socially appropriate or has she lost her social filters? Social filters keep people from touching people or objects without permission, saying inappropriate things, cursing or swearing, or taking off their clothes in public.

- Is she able to initiate social activity? Often as someone loses more cognitive capacity, it becomes more difficult to initiate social activity.

- Is she able to function well in group activities? Does being in small or large groups cause your loved one to become more anxious or agitated?

- Does taking her out of her residential community or home cause anxiety or agitation? For example, does she get anxious in the days and hours leading up to a trip or outing? Is she uncomfortable and restless in a new environment?

As you keep these answers in mind, the "Dementia Abilities Continuum" is a tool that I created to help families understand common patterns of dementia and the disease progression.

Dementia Abilities Continuum

The Dementia Abilities Continuum can help families assess where their loved one might be with their dementia and what symptoms to expect. This continuum has three stages, which are meant as a general guide and not as absolutes. At different points in your loved one's illness, he may vacillate between one stage and another.

Mostly-Abled

In this first stage, your loved one most likely will have difficulty with short-term memory. It is common for her to be aware of these memory challenges and try to cover them up. It is not unusual for a person to become less aware of her cognitive and physical decline. This in turn can make it more difficult for her to accept help or to consider moving into a facility. You might notice the following symptoms:

- More forgetfulness than usual. She might misplace items more frequently, repeatedly ask the same question and not remember what has been said to her.

- More confusion.

- More difficulty with focusing.

- Struggling with tasks she was always able to accomplish, such as failing to keep up with bank accounts, bills or taxes.

- Struggling with finding the correct word.

- Experiencing feelings of embarrassment or shame from not remembering a familiar person's name.

- Beginning to withdraw from social functions, especially those in which she used to participate.

- Compensating for memory problems by trying to change the topic or by answering a question in a more generalized way.

For example, if asked how long she has lived in her home, instead of saying "30 years," she might say, "for a long time."

- Experiencing some paranoia, for example, accusing you or others of taking her money or jewelry.

Less-Abled

During this second stage, your loved one's long-term memory will become more impaired and her cognitive skills become more compromised. She may also begin to have some physical issues with balance, walking, and perception. She may have bladder incontinence. She may experience more confusion with performing her "activities of daily living" or ADL's, such as bathing, dressing, grooming, and food preparation. Her personal hygiene may suffer, along with her ability to stay properly nourished and maintain a clean and safe home environment. Some examples include:

- Being increasingly forgetful and unaware that she is not remembering, or asking the same questions over and over.

- Becoming more easily and more frequently confused. She may forget how to use the remote control or even get lost while driving to familiar places.

- Needing reminders to take a shower or change stained or dirty clothes.

- Having more difficulty with her attention span and following directions.

- Substituting the wrong word and jumbling her words in sentences.

- Beginning to lose some of her long-term skills and functioning. For example, she may not be able to remember easy tasks, such as how to follow a recipe or how to fix things in the house.

- Forgetting family members' names or details about her past.

- Having more difficulty with sitting still.

- Needing more supervision around safety. For example, your loved one might leave the stove on or have spoiled food in the refrigerator. She might make impulsive decisions due to an inability to think through the consequences, such as letting a stranger in the house.

Un-abled

At this third stage, your loved one's symptoms of dementia are quite severe. She now requires complete help with her ADLs and cannot function without continual supervision. The following typically characterize this stage:

- Mainly communicates through body language.

- Not aware of time, place or person.

- Being incontinent of bladder and bowel.

- Having more difficulty with eating and swallowing.

- Having more health problems, such as frequent infections. Urinary Tract Infections (UTIs) are particularly common due to incontinence.

- Not being able to walk, either needing to be in a wheel chair or recliner.

- Becoming bed-ridden.

In Summary

Understanding your loved one's abilities and strengths can help you identify more meaningful ways to be together. Assessing which stage your loved one is in can help you know what to expect, as well as help you engage most appropriately. The next chapter will offer tips and ideas about how to spend the best possible time with one another, regardless of the stage of dementia.

Chapter 2

How to Visit with a Loved One who has Dementia

> "All people, including those with dementia, need the opportunity to give and receive affection and enjoy companionship of others."
>
> -Rethinking Alzheimer's Care

VISITING with a loved one with dementia can be a positive experience. This chapter provides some tips on how to improve your visits, as well as discusses some of the common challenges that can arise with dementia. I would like to begin with some common questions care partners have asked about visiting their loved one in a residential community. Keep in mind, however, that many of the tips also apply to visiting with someone who lives in his own home. My responses reflect my observations and experiences from years of practice.

Commonly Asked Questions

How often should I visit?

The frequency of visitation depends on many factors, such as the relationship you have with your loved one; how far away you live; your own family or work responsibilities; and your own health needs. Some care partners visit daily, while others visit several times a week. One to two visits a week is generally the norm when living in the same area. Remember that the quality of the visit is much more important than how often you visit.

How often should I visit if I just placed my spouse in a residential facility?

In my experience, spouses tend to feel tremendous guilt about placing their husband, wife or partner into a residential community, and then feel pressure to visit quite frequently. When your spouse first moves into a residential community, it is not unusual to want to visit every day. If you do, I recommend keeping the visit to 1 to 1 ½ hours. After a few weeks, I usually suggest that you try not to visit every day. One of the most important goals for spouses is to let the facility caregivers get to know your loved one and trust that they will properly care for him or her. In addition, it is important to work with the staff so that they learn what is most important to your loved one.

How long should the visit be?

How much time you spend with your loved one largely depends on how receptive your loved one is to your visit. As a general rule, I typically recommend no more than 1 to 1 ½ hours. If your loved one has significant cognitive challenges, less time may be better.

Is there a best time to visit?

Generally it is best to visit earlier in the day. Be mindful that people with dementia can experience more agitation and confusion towards the end of the day. Whenever possible, also try to visit on different days, such as, on the weekends when staffing is lower and there may be fewer activities.

Is it ok NOT to visit?

Yes, it is certainly okay not visit. Care partners need time away to replenish, whether it is time off or a vacation.

Is it ok to take a vacation?

Yes. It is perfectly acceptable to want and take a vacation, even though many care partners are afraid or feel guilty about doing so. If you go away, I suggest establishing an emergency back-up plan. While you are away, consider having someone, perhaps a grandchild or friend, who can be available if something happens, such as a fall or acute medical condition. You can also hire a home care agency to be on call if needed.

Should I expect my visits to always be good?

No, it is not realistic to expect your visits will always be positive. Due to neurological changes in the brain, people with dementia can behave very differently day to day. So be kind and gentle, and don't blame yourself for an unfulfilling visit. Hopefully the next time you visit will be a more positive experience.

Tips for Positive Visits

Now that we have discussed when and how often to visit, here are some general tips for making the visit more positive.

- Try to visit when your loved one is at her best. Keep track of your visits and note how comfortable or uncomfortable your loved one was when you visited. Consider asking the staff for their recommendations about the best time to visit.

- Whenever possible, visit your loved one during a community activity, such as a musical, art or entertainment program.

- Bring someone with you. This can be enjoyable for your loved one and takes some of the focus off of you. Children and animals are also wonderful visitors and can enhance everyone's time together.

- Arrange to visit your loved one along with another resident. Again, this takes the focus off just the two of you and can help encourage new connections for your loved one and the other resident.

- Ask a friend or family member to visit your loved one instead. It's good for both of you. It allows for you to take a break, and it's nice for your loved one to have other people with whom to interact.

- Pay attention to the environment during your visit. Busy, noisy environments can be overwhelming and very distracting. Whenever possible, find a space in the community that is quiet and has minimal distractions.

- Recognize how your spirit and mood impact the visit. Your loved one can very quickly sense how you are feeling. Try not to visit when you are tired, rushed or feel particularly ambivalent about being there.

Behavioral Expressions and Other Common Challenges

Dementia can cause neurological changes in a person's brain, which can result in memory loss, confusion and disorientation. This in turn, can cause misunderstanding and lead to "behavioral expressions." Behavioral expressions refer to the actions that are an attempt to *communicate a need*. Behavioral expressions are especially common when a person loses the ability to verbally communicate. For example, a person might start pacing because she needs to use the restroom. Or a person might become agitated because she doesn't feel well. The following are some common behavioral expressions and some suggestions on how to handle them. Keep in mind that these behaviors may occur during one visit, but not the next. They are not predictable, so being flexible is a must!

Pacing and Wandering

Some people with dementia might pace or walk continually throughout the day. If your loved one tends to pace on a more regular basis, don't try to stop the behavior. This behavior might be neurological. Perhaps you can sing with him or try pointing out things of interest while walking together. However, sometimes pacing occurs because something is bothering him. He might be in pain, need to go to the restroom or is too hot or too cold.

Frequent Distractions

When people with dementia progress in their illness, they can become more easily and frequently distracted. If this applies to your loved one, start by evaluating the environment. Is the environment noisy, bustling with people; is the room temperature comfortable? If there is nothing obvious in the physical environment, try to establish eye contact or get her attention by gently touching her hand, shoulder or leg. Sometimes, you can try engaging her in an activity like working on a puzzle, and then see if she can follow along. Lastly, you might see if you can just sit quietly and hold hands.

Excess Sleeping

As a person's dementia progresses, it is not unusual for him to sleep an excessive amount. If this is occurring with your loved one, find out if your loved one is sleeping through the night, or if medications could be a factor. If neither of those is a concern, it may be that this is the new normal. If your loved one is sleeping while you are visiting, consider being present by holding his hand or gently massaging his neck or shoulders. You can also softly read or talk to him or listen to soothing music.

Sundowning

Sundowning is the term that describes a set of behaviors that can occur later in the afternoon or early evening as the sun goes down – hence the name, "sundowning." With sundowning, a person experiences more agitation, anxiety and confusion at the end of the day. If this happens with your loved one, try to visit at another time. Let the staff at the community care for your loved one in the evening, as they have experience with this phenomenon.

Agitation

Agitation can result from dementia or may be caused by something else. If your loved one is agitated on a regular basis, inform the staff so they can monitor the situation. See if you or the staff can determine any environmental, medical or physical reasons for the agitation. If so, alleviating the cause may decrease the agitation. Keep in mind that some people may need medication to control the agitation. It can be difficult to visit a loved one when he is agitated. If you are not able to calm your loved one down, it might be best to visit with him another time.

Asking to Go Home

Dementia can impact a person's understanding of his situation. When your loved one lives in a residential community, he may ask to go home because he may not remember or be aware of where he is. Your goal should be to calm him down, and at the same time, validate his concern. You might want to consider saying, "I know you want to go home" and then try talking about old memories of home. For example, talk about what the home looked like, about the neighbors or the environment around the home. Or try to change the topic altogether. Ultimately, if a person with dementia has the opportunity for more meaningful engagement, the desire to go home can diminish.

In Summary

My hope is that you are now armed with some general knowledge about visiting. The next chapter will introduce the concepts of meaningful engagement and person-centered activities, so you can experience more pleasant time together.

Chapter 3

♥

Meaningful Engagement and Person-Centered Activities

> "If a man is given two pennies,
> he should spend one to buy a
> loaf of bread and with the other,
> a flower to make life worth living"
>
> A Chinese Proverb

ALL people need meaningful engagement to keep their mind, body and spirit alive and well. In addition, we yearn to feel connected to people and to the world around us. When your loved one is diagnosed with dementia, you may struggle with how to stay connected. The purpose of this chapter is to introduce the concepts of *meaningful engagement and person-centered activities*, which are vitally important to your loved one's self-esteem and well-being.

Meaningful Engagement

Meaningful engagement refers to the process of assessing your loved one's capabilities and providing an opportunity for your loved one to engage with you and others in pleasurable ways. For instance, if she is able to follow and understand conversation, then you can still talk and share information in many of the same ways you always have. However, if your loved one is having difficulty with conversations, you may need to share less information and possibly find other ways to communicate. For example, you might look at old pictures together, sing songs or listen to music.

My Story

When I reflect on the 14 years that I visited my mother at the nursing home, meaningful engagement was dependent mostly *on me*, not my mother. I had to step back and be mindful of how to adapt to my mother's abilities, so that I could find new and different ways to be together. This required that I had to meet my mother where she was cognitively, emotionally and physically. I had to recognize the way we spent time together would need to change, which meant I had to be open to different ways of being together. At first this took me out of my comfort zone. I was not one to be spontaneous, but my mother loved dancing and singing at a moment's notice. So when I did that with her, it turned out to be a lot of fun for the both of us!

I also learned to ask other people to join us, taking some of the focus off the two of us. In addition to her cognitive decline, I had to adjust to her physical decline. In the later stages of her dementia, my mother was no longer able to sit up comfortably and was in bed a great amount of the day. Instead of sitting next to her, I decided, what the heck, I would get in bed with her! We would lie side by side, singing or humming or just holding hands. That special time is still embedded in my heart.

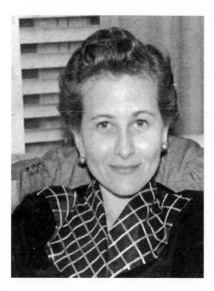 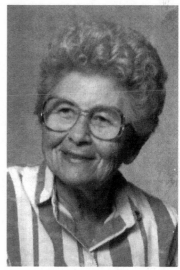

I share the above to provide some food for thought. Ultimately, you will have to find your own way to engage. And let me add, this may take experimenting and learning from some mistakes. It can't be said enough that meaningful engagement requires patience, flexibility and a willingness to plan your visits. Once you are able to accomplish this, you will be amazed at how much easier it can be to create a new, enjoyable and meaningful relationship.

Person-Centered Activity

Person-centered activity involves providing activities that are based on your loved one's past or present interests, hobbies, work history, family or spiritual life. Creating person-centered activities requires learning to match the activities to your loved one's abilities. This increases the likelihood that your loved one can engage in an activity with more ease. Person-centered activities also reinforce the notion that your loved one's life can still hold meaning and value.

♥

Mary's Story

Mary had been moved into assisted living with memory care because she was requiring more help and supervision due to her dementia. Her focus and communication skills were limited, and she was increasingly forgetful. Mary had been an editor for a large, well respected publishing house, and valued using her words. Losing her cognitive ability left her depressed. She was having a difficult time adjusting to these changes. On one visit, she clearly articulated, "I feel like I have been demoted." She felt that everyone in memory care was "stupid," and that the staff treated her that way as well. Recognizing that she was still able to read, I suggested to the activities director that Mary be given the opportunity to read to the residents. She needed an activity that would help preserve her self-esteem. The activity director arranged for Mary to read poetry and short stories several times a week to the residents. She loved it. It was remarkable to see the restoration of her self-esteem and the pleasure she derived from this activity. Additionally, she was given the task for making sure the books in their library were in good order. These activities held tremendous meaning for Mary and helped her feel "less stupid."

Dr. K's Story

As Dr. K. aged, he developed dementia believed to be related to years of head trauma from football. As his cognitive and physical abilities declined, he had to move into a nursing home. Yet in spite of his condition, he was proud of being a physician and still believed he was practicing medicine. Creating person-centered activities required that he be given a job that helped him feel as if he was still practicing. He was made the "medical director" of the nursing home. His family brought his white coat, gave him his stethoscope, and the staff made him a "chart." They sat him at a nearby desk and would occasionally ask him a medical question. Remarkably, he was often right on track with the answer. Everyone knew him affectionately as Dr. K. and Dr. K. happily thought he was the director of the unit!

Jake's Story

Jake was living in a memory care community and insisted on wearing his winter coat-- even in 80-degree weather. For many years in his youth, he had delivered the paper in rural Idaho. I had a notion that he was living back during that time of his life. I suggested to the activity director that he be given a "paper route." To do so, the staff collected old papers, wrapped them with a rubber band, and gave them to Jake. Each morning he delivered the papers to the residents' rooms. Caregivers would then collect them and give them back to him, so he could deliver them again in the late afternoon. He delivered papers two times a day with gusto and pride, as he had in the past. His behavioral expressions lessened some as he was able to engage in this more person-centered activity.

Benefits of Meaningful Engagement

I hope these examples were helpful and will inspire you to give this approach a try! There are many benefits to meaningful engagement and person-centered activities.

For Your Loved One

- Strengthens self-esteem

- Relieves boredom

- Offers meaningful socialization and connection

- Helps one to sleep better

- Lessens loneliness and depression

- Preserves abilities

- Helps organize the day

- Connects one to her past

- Helps one remain connected to others

For Care Partners

- Gain insights about your loved one which you may have not thought about before

- Experience a different side of your loved one that brings you joy

- Learn more about yourself, especially when you allow yourself to open to new experiences

- Develop more compassion and perhaps even a deeper love or understanding for your loved one

- Recognize that there are many non-verbal ways to communicate that can be quite powerful and meaningful

- Appreciate being more in the moment and being together

In Summary

Keeping your loved one connected, engaged and as active as possible is extraordinarily important to well-being. It helps her feel as if her life still matters. And you most likely will discover the benefits for you as well!

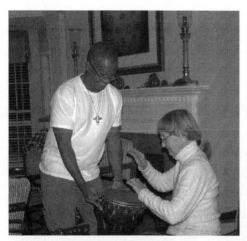
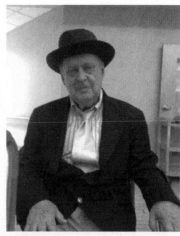
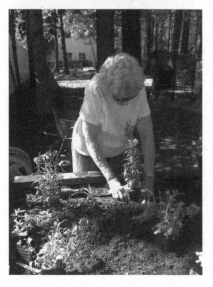
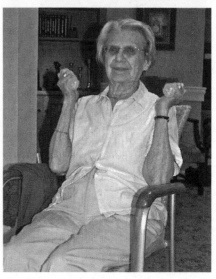

Chapter 4

Creating Person-Centered Activities

Find new ways to engage with
your loved one. Connecting to
your loved one's spirit helps
keep your relationship alive

CREATING person-centered activities requires staying open to new ways of being together with your loved one and is not as difficult as it may seem at first. In some ways, creating person-centered activities is akin to making a special meal for your loved one. You find a recipe he likes, purchase the ingredients, gather the proper utensils and prepare the food. Then hopefully you and your loved one enjoy eating the meal together. This chapter discusses the basic principles of person-centered activities, as well as describes different categories of activities. Within each category, there are suggestions for specific activities and the needed supplies, as well how to adapt the activities to meet your loved one's changing cognitive needs.

Principles of Person-Centered Activities

The overall goal of a person-centered activity is to find ways to be together that enhance enjoyment for you and your loved one. When considering person-centered activities, there are some basic principles to keep in mind.

Identify your loved one's interests.

When someone has dementia, learning new activities or hobbies can be quite difficult and even impossible for many. It's best to consider activities that have been lifelong interests. For example, if your loved one enjoyed flowers, flower arranging might be a fun activity. Or if your loved one enjoyed fixing things, you could bring items that he could take apart and put back together.

Be the Initiator.

People with dementia can lose their ability to plan activities. This means that you, as the care partner, will have to initiate the activity.

Assess your loved one's abilities and skills.

It's important to match activities with your loved one's abilities; otherwise, he could get easily frustrated or lose interest. For example, if his attention span is short, then gear the activity to 10 to 15 minutes. Or, if he can no longer track your conversation, consider listening to music instead of trying to engage him in conversation.

Ensure activities are adult in nature.

The dignity of the person should always be considered. For example, find puzzles or coloring books designed for adults. Those created for children can be demeaning and therefore upsetting to your loved one.

Stimulate as many of the senses as possible.

Try activities that use a combination of senses, such as sight, sound, smell, taste and touch. When someone has dementia, his attention span may become more limited, which is why using other senses can help. Use a few different ones, which can facilitate connection to the activity. For example, if your loved one enjoyed baseball, bring a leather mitt to feel and smell, a baseball to hold and touch, hot dogs to smell and taste, and then either sing or play "take me out to the ball game." You can also look at pictures of favorite baseball players.

Encourage spiritual or religious connection.

If your loved one is a spiritual or religious person, try to identify activities that are familiar and comforting. This could be reading passages from the Bible, listening to religious or spiritual music or reciting some prayers together.

Adapt activities over time.

Be mindful that the ways that you engage will depend on where your loved one is on the dementia continuum. Over time, you may need to change what you can do.

Introduction to Activities

The heart remembers

Discovering new ways to engage with a loved one with dementia can help remove much of your fear and apprehension. The goal of spending positive time together is being able to connect spirt to spirit and heart to heart. Just because a loved one loses some of her cognitive abilities does mean that she loses her ability to connect to her spirit and heart. My hope is that this chapter will encourage meaningful connections.

There are lots of different activities that can be used to engage your loved one and I have tried to classify them into different categories such as life profession, hobbies or music. In subsequent pages, each category is described in more detail, along with different ideas on how you can implement the concepts within that category. In addition, there are suggestions for items and supplies to help you accomplish the activity. Some people may find it helpful to bring a laptop or tablet with them. The device can be used to search for information related to your loved one's hobby, such as looking at photography sites. Likewise, finding and playing songs or videos related to her favorite musician, for example, can be a great way to connect. The main objective is to have fun and to enjoy your time together.

With each of the ideas, consider what is most familiar to your loved one and what will bring him the most joy. There are many enjoyable activities that involve creative expression, such as cooking, music, crafts or gardening. Regardless of the activity, try tapping into different senses - taste, touch, smell, hearing and sight. Stimulating the senses can uplift your loved one's spirit and help her feel more connected. Make sure you scale the activity based upon your loved one's abilities. To help with this, each activity concludes with advice on how to adapt the activity to the three levels of ability described in the Dementia Abilities Continuum. Remember, the goal is to try to ensure that your loved one has a successful and enjoyable experience, no matter his cognitive ability. My hope is that you will discover new ways to engage with your loved that are meaningful to you both.

Activity Categories

─────────────────── ♥ ───────────────────

Life Profession Activities   Page 32

Activities that tap into past occupations or skills

Cultural Activities   Page 34

Celebrations that honor holidays, heritages, rituals and birthplaces

Reading Activities   Page 36

Stories, books and magazines can be read together

Gardening Activities   Page 38

Garden activities either inside or outside of your loved one's home or community

Cooking Activities   Page 40

Preparing or finding recipes that you can cook together

Music Activities   Page 42

Listen to or sing music that your loved one would enjoy

Creative Craft Activities   Page 44

Catch-all category for creative outlets such as mosaics, paper flowers, painting flower pots

Hobby Activities

Using past interests, such as stamp collecting or fishing, to engage your loved one

Special Interests Activities

Tapping into unique interests, such as movie stars, to being a civil war history buff

Physical Activities

Exercises specifically adapted for those with dementia

Pets & Animals Activities

Activities that foster interaction with animals such as dogs and cats

Intergenerational Activities

Interaction with children and young adults

Social Activities

Activities that foster interaction between several individuals

Activities of Daily Living

Daily living tasks such as nail care, shaving, or putting on makeup

Life Profession Activities

This category is very person-centered depending on your loved one's profession, occupation or life skills. The ideas can foster reminiscence and remind people with dementia of their contribution to family, friends, past colleagues and the community. Furthermore, the tasks associated with this category can be retained for a significant time in long-term memory.

Ideas

- Invite former colleagues or work associates to visit and spend time with your loved one

- When possible, show pictures or make a road trip to the old workplace

- Bring in some of the tools of the trade and reminisce with them, whether they were equipment, books or other items

- Bring in photo albums or pictures of your loved one participating in his occupation

Examples of Questions to Ask

- What was your life's work? A particular profession? Homemaker?

- Where did you work?

- What was your first job?

- Do you remember how much you got paid?

- If you were a homemaker, what did you enjoy most?

Items to Consider

- Tools and utensils that were used by your loved one

- Books or videos about the occupation or life skill he participated in

- Tablet to look up the information about her workplace or occupation

Adapting the Life Profession Activity - School Teacher Example

More-abled: Think of ways to help her reminisce about what it was like teaching. You can use the internet to look up pictures and other information about her school. Find out if she had a school yearbook, has any letters from former students or families that you could gather into a book for reminiscing. Talk about what it was like to be a school teacher and share how things have changed. If any of her students are still nearby, invite them to visit.

Less-abled: Tell her what you know about her being a school teacher. Perhaps there are special stories she might still remember when you share them with her. Bring in school supplies that she may have used when she was teaching. Look for books that have pictures of school children. Especially interesting can be looking at school children from around the world.

Un-abled: Tell her how many children loved her as a teacher. Perhaps share a few stories about her interaction with her students. Sing songs about school days.

Cultural Activities

This category is rich with all kinds of possibilities to keep your loved one connected to people and cultural activities that have been meaningful over the years. Too often people with dementia lose a sense of who they were and are. Spending time reminiscing can help your loved one hold on to her self-esteem. You can focus on celebrating and honoring your loved one's birthplace, rituals, heritage or holidays.

Examples of Questions to Ask

Birthplace

- When were you born?
- Where you were born?
- How long did you live there?

Family

- Do you have siblings?
- Where were they born?
- Can you tell me who these relatives are? (show pictures)

Heritage

- What heritage do you most identify with?
- When did you or your loved one's family come to this country?
- What particular customs honor your heritage?
- Are there certain religious beliefs that go along with your heritage?

Personal and National Pastime Rituals

- Which holidays held special meaning and how were they celebrated?

- Were there particular foods that you would eat?

- How were major events (birthdays, graduation) celebrated?

- Were there blessings or prayers that held special meaning?

- What music do you remember from your culture, heritage or religion?

Items to Consider

- Photographs or photo albums of the family

- Portable device to look up information

- Words to familiar holiday songs

- Blessings or prayers to say together

- Ritual items, such as prayer books, candle or a flag

- Foods that are associated with particular holidays, celebrations or events

Adapting the Activity: Celebrating a Birthday

Most-abled: Celebrate your loved one's birthday by taking him to his favorite restaurant. Consider inviting others.

Less-abled: If you take your loved one out for a meal, make sure the place is not overstimulating. Consider picking up his favorite food and celebrating with a small group of familiar people.

Un-abled: It's best to bring the celebration to him. Keep it simple and minimize the stimulation. Perhaps bring one food item and have just a few people present.

Reading Activities

Many people enjoy reading, and that is still true for people with dementia. Find topics that are of interest to your loved one, whatever that may be. This list of potential topics is endless: inspirational stories, history, cars, cooking, gardening, pets, famous people, or sports. Reading together can be comforting and enjoyable. Also, books that have pictures are highly encouraged as they can help keep your loved one more focused. As your loved one's cognitive abilities decline, you may have to read from magazines or short stories, or pick out parts from a book.

Ideas

- Read books or play audio books
- Read newspaper or magazine articles
- Read short stories or essays
- Read poems, limericks or famous sayings
- Read some old children's nursery rhymes
- Read Bible stories or verses
- Find picture books and look at them together
- Use interactive books
- Look through high school yearbooks
- Have a grandchild or young child read to your loved one

Items to Consider

- Books or audio books

- Magazines or newspapers

- Short story or essay collections

- Books of poetry, limericks, sayings or nursery rhymes

- Picture books

- Interactive books

- Yearbooks or other books with specific meaning for your loved one

Adapting the Reading Activity

More-abled: You can bring a book that would appeal to your loved one. It might be a book on presidents, history, science or even fiction. You can read sections or chapters together, and then discuss the content.

Less-abled: Make sure you bring a book or magazine that has fewer words and more pictures. You can read to your loved one or look through the pictures. Limericks and rhyming poems are great fun to read.

Un-abled: Identify and read passages, poems or even nursery rhymes that have been familiar to your loved one.

Gardening Activities

Gardening can be very therapeutic for your loved one and can help engage several different senses. In addition, gardening can bring back memories for those who had gardens or farms. Plants and flowers can be used for decorations, celebrations or just because they look and smell nice. Make sure that any plants you use are non-poisonous. (There is a list of non-poisonous plants on the National Alzheimer's website.) Gardening is also a wonderful activity for children to participate in with your loved one.

Ideas

- Bring in cut flowers for centerpiece decorations

- Decorate pots or garden markers

- Bring house plants into your loved one's room and water them together

- Plant seeds in small cups and watch them grow

- Create an herb box garden in your loved one's apartment or room

- Plant flowers, herbs or vegetables at your loved one's residence

- Engage children to help plant a garden at your loved one's residence

- Plant seasonal flowers in outside pots or garden areas

- Volunteer you and your loved one to help water plants at the residential community

- Look through picture books of flowers or garden magazines

Items to Consider

- Cut flowers and a vase
- Supplies to decorate pots, such as stickers, buttons, shells, markers and paint
- House plants, flowers or herbs
- Planting supplies, such as gardening soil, plants, seeds and a watering can
- Small cups for seed starting
- Gardening magazines or books

Adapting the Gardening Activity

More-abled: Your loved one should be able to help with planting seeds, herbs, vegetables or flowers. She can taste, touch or smell some of the plants. If she grew something, consider using some of the harvested herbs or vegetables in a recipe. You can also talk about the past, and what she planted in her garden. Consider bringing some gardening books for her to look through.

Less-abled: Your loved one most likely can still help with simple tasks, such as planting vegetables or flowers in a pot. She can taste, touch or smell some of the flowers, herbs or vegetables. You can reminisce by asking questions about her gardening, or remind her of what she planted over the years. Perhaps you can show her some pictures of her garden.

Un-abled: Your loved one might be able to enjoy smelling flowers, or even tasting vegetables or herbs. She is not likely to be able to help with planting.

Cooking Activities

Cooking can be a fun activity and can be active or passive. Your loved one can help with cooking, talk about cooking, savor the smells, or enjoy eating what you made. If this is not possible, she can just be with you while you cook. The ideas below require minimal effort and can be easily done with portable cooking tools.

Ideas

- Make a simple recipe of one her favorite foods
- Look through cooking magazines or cookbooks together
- Write down favorite recipes to pass down to others
- Bake bread in a bread maker
- Bake cookies or cupcakes in a small toaster oven
- Make pancakes or French toast in an electric skillet
- Make waffles in a waffle maker
- Blend up frozen smoothies
- Make ice cream or frozen yogurt in an ice cream maker
- Stir fry in an electric wok or skillet
- Make juices in a blender
- Cook chili, stews or other recipes in a slow cooker

Examples of Questions to Ask

- Which were your favorite foods to cook or bake?
- What were your family's favorite recipes?
- Did she ever bake something her mother had made?
- Have you passed along recipes to other family members?
- Have the recipes changed over the years? How?

Items to Consider

- Familiar recipes
- Cookbooks or magazines
- Electric skillet or wok
- Toaster oven or slow cooker
- Bread maker
- Waffle iron
- Blender or juicer
- Ice cream maker

Adapting the Cooking Activity - A Favorite Recipe

More-abled: Invite your loved one to help make one of her favorite recipes, such as a simple dessert. Reminisce about how cooking has changed over her lifetime. After the dessert is made, enjoy eating it together.

Less-abled: Determine how much your loved one can participate in making her favorite recipe. You may need to help her remember what desserts she enjoyed and remind her of the ingredients. She most likely will enjoy eating whatever you have made together.

Un-abled: Most likely you will need to make the recipe. Consider having your loved one sit with you while you bake. Share how much you enjoyed her dessert and other things she made. Hopefully, your loved one can enjoy smelling, tasting or eating what you have made.

Music Activities

For people with dementia, music is retained in the brain a long time. In fact, even those who have trouble communicating verbally can often still sing the words to songs. Music stimulates the brain and can help encourage conversation, foster activity, and even ease people during showers, dressing and grooming. In addition, music helps people feel connected.

Try to find music that is familiar to your loved one. This could be music from different decades or familiar genres, such as country, jazz, pop, or classical. Also consider bringing in rhythmic musical instruments to make your own music. Drumming is a great way to engage and have fun. Below is a list of different ways to bring music into your loved one's life.

Ideas

- Play instruments together
- Listen to music that is calming, spiritual or religious
- Watch music videos
- Sing or dance together
- Have a grandchild play a musical instrument for your loved one
- Look through books of famous singers and song writers

Items to Consider

- Musical instruments
  (drums, bells, tambourine, maracas or rain sticks)

- Portable device to watch music videos or listen to music

- Sheet music or words to songs

- Videos or books about famous singers and musicians

Adapting the Music Activity - Drumming Example

More-abled: Drum on two separate drums, or share one drum together. You can drum first and then encourage your loved one to drum next. Take turns back and forth, or try drumming to music.

Less-abled: Simplify the activity by having your loved one do simple hand movements on the drum. The two of you could take turns drumming, or you both can both drum together.

Un-abled: Don't expect your loved one to participate in drumming; instead, allow him to enjoy listening to or watching the drumming activity.

Creative Craft Activities

There are lots of simple crafts that can bring pleasure to you and your loved one. Listed below are a variety of ideas for crafts. I hope they stimulate different possibilities for you. Just a note: make sure that craft supplies are non-toxic and child-safe (with no sharp edges). Supervise closely if there are any items that could be eaten or swallowed.

Ideas

- Buy a wooden item to decorate, such as a door hanger or bird house
- Color together in adult themed coloring books
- Make holiday/birthday cards
- Make tissue flowers
- Make lavender herbal bags
- Decorate a favorite item, such as a picture frame, flower pot or stepping stone
- Make book or plant markers
- Make religious holiday decorations, such as wreaths, ornaments or hats
- Make trivets out of ice cream sticks
- Decorate clothing, such as visors or hats
- Make a theme-based collage from photos or magazine pictures

Items to Consider

- Craft store wooden objects
  (door hangers, picture frames, bird houses)

- Crayons, markers, colored pencils or non-toxic paint

- Adult coloring books

- Tissue paper

- Dried lavender and small cloth bags

- Decorations, such as stickers, glitter, buttons, shells,
  wood cut-outs

- Ice cream sticks

- Visors or straw hats

- Photos or magazine pictures

Adapting the Craft Activity - Decorating a Bird House

More-abled: Find a bird house that he can decorate using buttons, mosaic tiles, shells or whatever else you choose. Talk with your loved one about what the project means. For example, ask about the different types of birds he used to have in his yard. You can also look at different bird books.

Less-abled: Determine how much he can help decorate the bird house. Consider easy ways to decorate, such as using paint or non-toxic markers. Talk about the birds that were in his backyard and show him pictures of various birds.

Un-abled: Consider showing your loved one a bird house instead of decorating it. Perhaps you can take him outside to hang the bird house, or just sit and enjoy listening to the birds. You can remind him of the different birds he used to see.

Hobby Activities

Connecting to your loved one using hobbies should focus on his specific and unique interests. This could include cooking, stamp or coin collecting, gardening, model trains or any other cherished activity. The hobby you select should encourage reminiscing, reinforce self-esteem, and validate your loved one's life. Since there are so many possibilities, I will just provide an example using fishing. This is a fun topic to discuss and bring in the actual physical items.

Ideas

Fishing

- Bring in a tackle box to rummage through
- Bring a fishing pole and the lures
- Look through books and magazines on fishing
- Show pictures of past fishing trips
- Take your loved one on a fishing outing

Examples of Questions to Ask

- Where did you fish?
- What kind of fishing rod and bait did you use?
- What kind of fish did you catch?
- What was the largest fish you ever caught?
- Did you prepare your fish and cook it?
- What was your funniest or most favorite fishing memory?

Items to Consider

- Fishing rod
- Bait
- Tackle box
- Fishing hooks and lures
- Fishing magazines and books
- Pictures of fishing trips

Adapting the Hobby Activity - Fishing Example

More-abled: Take your loved one fishing. If you can't bring her fishing, consider bringing the tackle box and fishing rods to discuss. Or bring in fishing books, magazines or videos. Reminisce about fishing.

Less-abled: Perhaps you can have some fun by setting up a small children's wading pool and dropping in some fake fish to be 'caught' with a fishing net. You can reminisce with your loved one or pretend that you caught the same fish she used to catch in the past. Perhaps bring some pictures of the fish she used to catch.

Un-abled: Most likely your loved one will not be able to fish. Maybe you can just reminisce with her and share some fishing stories or sing some songs about fishing.

Special Interests Activities

Like hobbies, using special interests to connect to your loved one is very personal. Those interests could include movie stars, geography, ancient history, or any other topic that your loved one feels passionate about. Use her special interest as a way to encourage engagement and reminiscing. Since there are so many possibilities, I will just provide an example using movie stars.

Ideas

Movie Star

- Look through magazines or books on famous movie stars
- Watch short video clips
- Listen to the music of famous movie stars

Examples of Questions to Ask

- What was it like going to the movies in the olden days?
- How much did it cost?
- Who were your favorite movie stars?
- Did you ever dream of being a famous movie star?
- Do you remember when you first saw a famous movie star on TV? What movie or show was he/she in?
- What were your favorite movies or TV shows that your movie stars were in?
- Did you ever see a famous movie star in person?

Items to Consider

- Magazines

- Books

- Biographies

- Portable device to listen to or watch videos

Adapting the Special Interest Activity - Movie Star Example

More-abled: Identify a movie star that your loved one really likes, for example, Barbra Streisand. Look at some videos of her work. Play some of her music.

Less-abled: Bring some pictures of Barbra Streisand. Listen to some of her music and maybe sing some of her famous songs together.

Un-abled: Listen to some of your loved one's favorite Barbra Streisand music.

Physical Activities

Care partners sometimes forget about physical activity as a way to engage their loved one. It's a great way to be together and it's good for the mind, body and spirit! There are a variety of ways to have fun while engaging in modified forms of physical exercise. Just match the activity to your loved one's abilities. Consider adding music to keep the activity more interesting. If your loved one is more cognitively and physically disabled, the physical activity will need to be limited to gentle movements.

Ideas

- Exercise by waving scarves to music

- Walk either inside or outside together

- Play games, such as putt-putt or horse shoes

- Lift one or two pound weights

- Stretch to soothing music

- Use swim noodles to make circles or figure eights, which helps with range of motion

- Hit a balloon back and forth

- Toss different size/colored balls

Items to Consider

- Different colored scarves

- Sports equipment, such as horse shoes or indoor putting greens

- Light hand weights (no more than 1 or 2 pounds)

- Portable device that can stream music

- Exercise videos specifically designed for older adults

- Swim noodles

- Balloons

- Different size or types of balls (small balls, soft balls)

Adapting the Physical Activity - Waving Scarf Example

More-abled: Find different length or colored scarves. It's most fun to wave the scarf to music. Wave them separately or wave them together. Or use the scarves to dance together.

Less-abled: Adapting this activity requires a long scarf so that you lead the activity. Hold one end and encourage your loved one to hold the other end. Wave the scarf together. Again, music can make the activity a lot more fun.

Un-abled: If your loved one is not able to follow any directions, you will need to do most of the movement. Music can help keep some attention or focus. Try to do different motions together.

Pets & Animals Activities

This category can be very important to people with dementia, particularly if they have or had pets or enjoy animals. They can provide meaningful ways for people with dementia to connect without having to verbally communicate. Pets can bring much comfort and joy, and be a great way to foster interaction.

Ideas

- Bring a dog, cat or other animal to visit with your loved one
- Show pictures of the various pets that your loved one had enjoyed
- Look through magazines or books with dogs, cats or other animals
- View animal or pet videos on your portable device
- Share how people seem to pamper their pets
- Share stories about service dogs

Examples of Questions to Ask

- Did you have pets or farm animals growing up?
- What were the names of your animals?
- What kind of animals did you have?
- Where did the pets or animals live?
- Do you have any funny stories about your pet?

Items to Consider

- A dog, cat or animal that can visit your loved one

- Picture books or magazines of dogs, cats or other animals

- Portable device to show videos or look up pictures of animals

- Find and play TV shows that feature pets, animals or nature

Adapting the Pet Activity

More-abled: If your loved one either has had or enjoys dogs, bring a dog for a visit. She can walk the dog, show off the dog, or enjoy petting the dog. Another idea is to keep special treats in your loved one's residence, so she can give them to the dog.

Less-abled: Your loved one can still enjoy petting the dog, if she is not able to walk the dog. If you bring a lap dog, let her give the dog treats in her lap.

Un-abled: Your loved one might just enjoy seeing the dog, or if the dog is a lap dog, let the dog sit with her.

Intergenerational Activities

Children, teens and young adults can bring much joy to the lives of those living with dementia. Almost all of the activities described so far can also be done with young people. I encourage you to plan special visits with your loved one's grandchildren, great grandkids or other children he knows.

Ideas

- Sing together
- Do crafts together
- Read together
- Write poems together
- Exercise together
- Plant together
- Invite a young person to dance or sing for your loved one
- Cook together
- Look through magazines together

Items to Consider

- Song sheets
- Crafts supplies
- Books and magazines
- Paper and pencils or pens
- Cooking supplies
- Plants, pots and tools for planting

Adapting the Intergenerational Activity - Singing Example

More-abled: Bring along the words or song sheets, so that your loved one can follow along as the young person and your loved one sing together.

Less-abled: Determine how much your loved one can sing along, or if song sheets would be helpful. Try singing the words and encourage your loved one to sing a word or two, or even hum along.

Un-abled: Have the young person sing to your loved one.

Social Activities

Social activity is important for the mind, body and spirit of people with dementia. Research has demonstrated the importance of social interaction, as it can help create new neuron cells, stave off depression and help with anxiety. Many long-term care communities offer a variety of social activities that you can engage in with your loved one. Ask for their calendar. If your loved one is at home, think about setting up your own activity schedule. In either case, consider including others, such as other residents, friends and family, or someone from your loved one's spiritual community. It's a nice way to include others and it can take the focus off your loved one.

Ideas

In a Long-Term Care Community

- Visit during mealtime and share a meal
- Identify fun activities from the monthly calendar and visit during that activity
- Consider visiting your loved one with another resident
- Share a meal at your loved one's table with other residents

At Home

- Consider taking your loved one out to a museum or movie
- Arrange for friends to take him out
- Arrange for a social outing to visit with others
- Explore bringing your loved one to a day program for people with cognitive challenges
- Ask someone to take your loved one to spiritual services

Adapting the Social Activity - Meal Sharing Example

More-abled: Eating with your loved one can help him feel special and allows you to be introduced to his tablemates. This gives you an opportunity to get to know some of the other residents. Ask the tablemates questions, which can facilitate more interaction between you, your loved one and the others.

Less-abled: You may need to sit at the table and initiate the conversation if your loved one is having difficulty with social interaction. This can provide a wonderful opportunity to share information about your loved one and help facilitate more positive interaction with other residents.

Un-abled: At this stage, your loved one will most likely need help with eating. For some care partners, helping to feed a loved one can be an intimate way to connect. For others, this way can be too painful or uncomfortable. You have to decide what feels best.

Activities of Daily Living (ADLs)

When someone has dementia, he or she can forget to perform personal care, refuse to do it, or even refuse to allow others to help. ADLs are the day to day activities that your loved one used to do, such as nail care, shaving, fixing one's hair, polishing shoes, or putting on makeup. Regardless of your loved one's abilities, providing ADL care can be a nice way to connect.

Ideas

Female ADL Ideas

- Polish her nails

- Wash, set or comb her hair

- Apply makeup

- Massage her hands with nice smelling lotion

- Have fun with accessories, such as putting on scarves, hats or costume jewelry

- Have fun choosing outfits for special occasions

Items to Consider

- Nail polish
- Shampoo
- Brush or comb
- Hair curlers
- Manicure set

- Makeup
- Hand lotion
- Costume jewelry
- Scarves, hats and other clothes

Ideas

Male ADL Ideas

- Shave his face

- Put on aftershave lotion

- Shine his shoes

- File his finger nails and put on clear nail polish

- Try on different hats or ties

- Put on familiar smelling cologne

Items to Consider

- Shaving cream

- Aftershave lotion or cologne

- Shoe polish and cloth for shining shoes

- Nail clipper and nail file

- Clear nail polish

- Hats and ties

- Cologne

Adapting the Female ADL Activity - Makeup Example

More-abled: Bring all kinds of different makeup that your loved one can try putting on herself. Or have fun putting makeup on her or she can even try applying it to your face. You can ask when she first started using makeup and who taught her. Talk about how the makeup industry has become so big and how women use makeup to look younger.

Less-abled: Put makeup on your loved one and then show her how she looks. And of course, show her off to others!

Un-abled: Determine what your loved one will be comfortable with. Perhaps you can do something soothing like gently washing her hands or face. Consider using a warm wash cloth scented with a nice smell.

Adapting the Male ADL Activity - Shaving Example

More-abled: Bring in his favorite shaving supplies and allow him to shave his face, and then put on aftershave cologne. Perhaps reminisce about when he first shaved and who taught him.

Less-abled: Perhaps you can enjoy shaving your loved one. Bring in shaving cream, so he can smell it along with his after shave. You can remind him about how old he was when he first shaved and share stories about the first time you learned to shave.

Un-abled: Determine what your loved one will be comfortable with. You can wash his face and then consider putting on the aftershave he used to use. The smells can be comforting.

In Summary

Hopefully, you have increased awareness of the different ways you can spend time with your loved one. The key is to make sure the activities are meaningful and appropriate to his cognitive abilities. I have always shared with families that even though the brain might not remember, the heart does. Finding positive ways to be together can lift your loved one's spirit and help you feel more at ease.

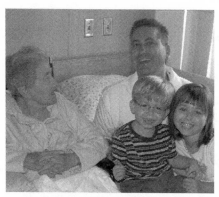

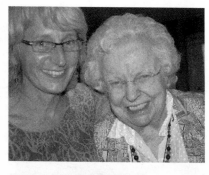

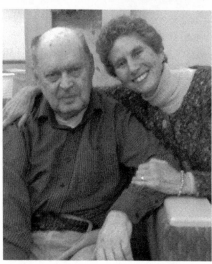

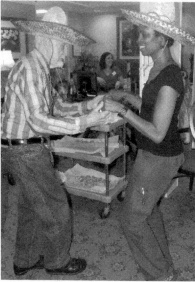

Chapter 5

Honoring Your Own Feelings

What truly make us human are our feelings. Embrace them, don't judge them

Do any of these statements sound familiar?

– "I love my mother, but am tired of visiting her every week."

– "I never was close with my father and am angry that I have to be the one to take care of everything!"

– "I have every good intention of a pleasant visit, but during our visit, she pushes my buttons and I leave feeling miserable."

– "I dread visiting; it always makes me sad."

Difficult Feelings

While this book focuses on positive ways to spend time with your loved one, I would be remiss if I didn't broach the topic of difficult feelings and how they can affect time spent with your loved one. Feelings are an integral part of you and cannot be easily pushed aside. It's important to get in touch with your feelings, *honor* them and try not to judge them. And remember, your feelings will be based upon your unique situation. I am going to focus on three feelings most frequently expressed by care partners – guilt, sadness and anger.

Guilt

At some point in the caregiving journey, care partners will experience some guilt. Guilt is an emotional response to a concern that you have about your loved one, and is a *normal feeling* no matter your past relationship. There are many reasons care partners can experience guilt: concern that you don't spend enough time with your loved one; feeling bad about moving a loved one who doesn't want or doesn't understand why he has to move; separating a couple who have been together for decades; or moving a loved one from his home into a residential community.

Guilt can also evoke other feelings, including regret or anger. Not addressing these feelings can make it much more difficult to accept whatever decision you make and can create more stress when you visit. Coping with guilt requires recognizing you did the *best* you could under the circumstances. When your guilt feelings arise, acknowledge them, remind yourself they are normal, and recognize that they may come and go every so often.

Kelly's Story

Kelly's mother was no longer able to live in her own home. Over the past five years, her mother was becoming more physically and cognitively frail. She had difficulty with many of her activities of daily living and seemed to be retreating more into herself. Kelly tried to support her mom at home, spending more and more time with her. Kelly's brother was very concerned about Kelly's well-being as well as his mother's. With continual prodding, he finally convinced Kelly to move their mother into an assisted living community. With tremendous guilt and a heavy heart, Kelly did so, and the guilt consumed her. She felt she needed to be at the assisted living community every day. Then to make matters worse, their mother took a bad fall and could only return to the assisted living community with 24/7 caregiver support. After one week of non-stop caregiver support, Kelly's guilt drove her to believe it was her job to take care of her mother. So she quit her job and went over to the assisted living community every day, staying eight to ten hours a day. Kelly was not aware of the emotional and physical toll it was taking on her. Kelly's brother became so concerned, he persuaded her to get some counseling. With my help, Kelly was able to see how her guilt was driving her to feel responsible for her mother's well-being. Kelly learned how to acknowledge her guilt, and then became aware of what was realistic in terms of spending time with her mother. She also learned that it wasn't the quantity of time spent with her mother, but the quality. I was able to give Kelly some new ideas and ways she could visit with her mother that were more fulfilling for them both.

Sadness

Sadness or sorrow is another emotion care partners may experience. Much of the sadness may have to do with recognizing that your relationship with your loved one has changed. And seeing your loved one lose more cognitive abilities can certainly conjure up a sense of loss of the past and for what is to come. These feelings are what professionals label as *anticipatory grieving*. Anticipatory grieving is acknowledging the sadness and grief you feel each time your loved one loses more abilities and independence. Some care partners describe it as losing your loved one in "little bits." Others describe anticipatory grieving as the "long goodbye." One of the greatest challenges care partners face is learning to let go of longing for how things used to be. It can be upsetting to realize that you can no longer have the same type of conversation or do the same things together. Admitting that your loved one has changed takes courage. You have to embrace these changes so you can focus on the remaining strengths. When you are able to do this, you will be better able to feel more at ease.

Lynne's Story

Lynne had been married to Ralph for almost 50 years. They had always been close and shared and enjoyed many of the same interests. They traveled a lot together and particularly loved spending time at their beach home. They didn't have children, but appreciated their many family members and friends. Their life was quite comfortable until out of nowhere, Ralph had a stroke. Fortunately for him, with intense therapy, he was able to make great strides towards his recovery. Yet despite the remarkable progress, Ralph had some serious residual effects that impacted him both physically and cognitively. Ralph was no longer able to live in the same home with Lynne because of his physical disabilities. And the stroke did change their relationship. Lynne could no longer depend on Ralph to take care of things in their home. Plus, Lynne had to now make the decisions that the two of them used to make together. Getting used to the "new normal" has been upsetting to both of them. Lynne has tremendous sadness as she feels that even though her husband is still living, she has lost "Ralph" as she knew him. Learning to let go of yearning for things to be the same takes a great amount of courage.

Ralph is struggling with not understanding why he can't continue to live his life like he used to. He isn't able to understand how his physical and cognitive impairments have impacted his ability to make appropriate or safe decisions. This creates tremendous anger for Ralph, which he directs at Lynne and results in additional sadness for Lynne. When Lynne acknowledged her sadness, and realized it is part of the grieving process, she was able to cope with her situation with less angst.

Anger

Anger is an emotion that is one of the most uncomfortable for care partners. Anger often arises from coping with your loved one's condition, which can include recognizing that your life has changed and that you cannot fix the situation. And there are some care partners that resent having to take care of their loved one. Anger is usually a *warning sign* that you are defending against the situation in which you have found yourself. In order to cope with anger, you have to first admit that you are angry. Then you have to determine whether it's worth holding on to your anger or recognizing that it may be healthier for you to acknowledge it and then let it go.

Sarah's Story

I worked with a care partner, Sarah, who was continually angry with the staff because her mother, who lived in a memory care assisted living community, was not getting dressed before she went to the breakfast meal. When I asked Sarah why this upset her so, she said that it had always been important to her mother to dress up and put on makeup before she went down for breakfast. Sarah mentioned her mother was very vain about her appearance. She wanted the staff to honor that for her mother. Yet Sarah did not realize that her mother was now fighting the staff when they tried to dress her each morning. They found that it was best to let her mother stay in her night clothes until she was calmer and more awake. Sarah finally was able to let go of how things used to be which helped ease both her and her mother.

This situation is not too unlike others. Learn to choose your battles – it can give you more ease and help alleviate your anger. Holding on to anger can cause stress and depression, and it can deplete your spirit. If you are struggling to overcome anger and having trouble letting go, consider seeking professional support. Sometimes you can be too close to the situation and being able to move your feelings aside requires outside help.

Troubled Past Relationships

Being confronted with caring for a person when your past relationship was difficult or abusive, can engender a variety of mixed feelings. Caring for such a family member can cause tremendous conflict and anger. Because of the toxicity of the relationship, you might want to consider working with a professional. An objective outsider may be able to help you navigate your feelings, and set appropriate limits and boundaries.

Steve's Story

Steve's father was verbally and physically abusive and they never had a good relationship. His father wanted him to become a lawyer, but Steve did not want that for himself. When he was a young adult, his father cut him off. When his mother died, Steve was contacted by his father's physician, who expressed concern about his father living alone with dementia. Steve had mixed emotions about getting involved, but ultimately did so out of familial obligation. Steve's father wasted no time verbally abusing him again and accusing Steve of wanting to take his money. Steve quickly realized that he needed professional support. The counselor helped Steve set boundaries and find other service providers to help his father so he didn't have to be directly involved.

When care partners have had troubled past relationships, it is critical that they carefully determine how much they are going to be involved, if at all. Exploring this with a professional can be enormously helpful.

In Summary

While I have discussed some of the most common feelings experienced by care partners, there are certainly others that I have not addressed. My hope is that you allow yourself to *own all your feelings* and know they are a normal part of caring.

Chapter 6

Finding Ease with Your Loved One at the End of Life

The end of life can be a mixed blessing, a sacred time and a time marked by great sadness

WHEN a loved one is close to end of life, many care partners can find being with her rather daunting. During this time, your loved one may be less communicative, less responsive, and may sleep a great deal. It is also possible she may not remember who you are or even be aware of your presence. The idea of spending time with someone who is unresponsive may seem like an exercise in futility. There is no doubt that being with a loved one at end of life requires a different kind of visit. It involves embracing what I refer to as *a healing presence*.

Healing Presence

A healing presence is being with – instead of doing something for – your loved one. It necessitates a willingness to just be quiet and present with your loved one. You set aside your busy life so you can savor the quiet and calm. A healing presence can also offer a different level of awareness and helps you appreciate the *grace moments*. Grace moments are those special moments that can be missed when you are continually in motion. You learn to pay attention to the ordinary, which can take on extraordinary meaning. Let me provide a few examples of visiting with a healing presence.

Jim's Story

I am the care partner for an elder gentleman, Jim, who has no children or known relatives. He was the ultimate gentleman – kind, friendly, and respectful to everyone he met. He was beloved wherever he lived. Over years of visits, I engaged with Jim in many different ways. When the weather was nice, I took him outside to get fresh air and sunshine. We listened to the birds and smelled the flowers. On other visits, we listened to his favorite music. I read passages from the Bible, which was important to Jim. We talked about his treasured memories of serving in the Marine Corps. Sadly, during the writing of this book, Jim's physical and cognitive health significantly declined. Jim couldn't sit up in a wheel chair, and was either in a recliner chair or his bed. He was transitioning toward the end of life.

I needed to have a *different kind of visit* with Jim. I had to shift into becoming a healing presence. Some days, I pulled up a chair beside him, quietly said hello and told him who I was. Then I would begin to gently massage his neck and head. Often his eyes were closed. I recall one visit when I was massaging Jim's neck and head. He suddenly opened his eyes and surprised me by saying, "Oh, that feels so good!" Then he closed his eyes and went back to sleep. On other occasions, I gently held his hand, and quietly sang to him. I brought in a CD player and played some soothing music. I asked Jim's caregivers to make sure the CDs were playing and changed on a regular basis. I also brought in lavender cream that we all could use on his face, hands and feet. Lavender is a very soothing scent.

I learned to appreciate the moments of solitude and time I spent with Jim. These visits taught me to be grateful for this sacred time. My focus was truly on being a healing presence by just being with him.

Caroline's Story

Caroline's husband had Parkinson's disease and Alzheimer's. She was struggling with how to be with her husband near the end of his life. I introduced Caroline to the concept of visiting with a healing presence. Being able to spend as much time as possible with her husband was most important to her. Yet she wasn't sure how to do this without feeling overwhelmingly sad. When I asked what would help lessen her sorrow, she immediately said reading a book or listening to music. So, I suggested she find comforting books that she could read to him, as well as find soothing music. I also encouraged her to bring a chair from home and leave it in her husband's room so she could be more comfortable. She would sit with her husband, hold his hand and sometimes read to him or just read her own book. She mentioned how much she appreciated that gentle, quiet time with him. When her husband died, she was grateful for the opportunity to approach his end of life with a healing presence. She said she didn't realize that there could be comfort and satisfaction at the end of life.

Tips for Visiting at End of Life

My hope is that introducing some of the examples and ideas below will stimulate other ways you can connect to your loved one at the end of life.

Visiting with your loved one during the end of life should fit what feels best for your situation. In addition to the examples above, there are other ways to visit with your loved one. You can:

- Bring nice smelling lotions to massage your loved one's hands, shoulders and neck.

- Wash your loved one's face with a warm and nicely scented wash cloth.

- Spray lavender oil on your loved one's pillow. You can also purchase a lavender mister that keeps a continual scent in the environment.

- Listen to soothing music.

- Hire a music therapist who can play or sing special music.

- Ask your minister or a clergy professional to recite some prayers.

- Read passages from the Bible or a spiritual book that has special meaning for you both.

- If you are comfortable, lie in bed with your loved one.

Hospice Services

An important way to find more ease at the end of life can be through engaging *hospice care* services. The goal of hospice care is to help manage symptoms, provide comfort and support, and improve your loved one's quality of life. Hospice is not curative care, but *comfort care*. Typically, a team of professionals is assigned to care for your loved one. This usually includes a physician, social worker, chaplain, nurse, volunteer and caregiver. The team closely monitors your loved one's care and can be a life-line to you as well. Hospice services are available to people who are at the end stages of their illnesses, and can be provided in-home or at a long-term care facility.

When a loved one has dementia, it can be more difficult to determine when hospice care might be appropriate. Many other illnesses have clearly defined end of life symptoms, but dementia does not. Infact, research indicates that hospice services are not utilized nearly enough because it can be difficult to recognize end of life symptoms in people with dementia. If you have any doubt, hospice professionals can help you determine if hospice care would be helpful. I highly encourage you to contact hospice and speak to the intake professional. He or she can help you determine if your loved one may be appropriate for hospice care.

In Summary

As you face the end of your loved one's life, I hope you will be able to discover ways to visit that can be special and meaningful to you. I leave you with a quote that might be comforting to you.

"People die, but loves does not die. It is recycled from one heart, from one life, to another"

-Rabbi Harold Kushner, Living and Life that Matters

Grab & Go Activity Boxes

GRAB & GO Activity Boxes are a theme related collection of items that you use to engage your loved one when you visit. Each box should be tailored to your loved one's interests and contain objects related to a past interest or passion. Since the boxes are person-centered, they can be very helpful for enhancing your visit and increasing connection. Grab & Go Activity Boxes can be used as often as you like. You may try using one each time you visit or every once in a while. People with dementia may not remember from visit to visit, so consider bringing the box frequently.

You may also want to change out the items in the box, or create more than one box, depending on your time and interest. Creating these boxes can be great holiday and birthday presents. They can also be fun for children to help put together. Grab & Go Boxes are especially useful for visits by others, particularly if they are less familiar with your loved one's interests.

In addition to the Grab & Go Activity Box, you may want to consider bringing other items to help enrich the visit with your loved one. For example, you could bring a portable device to watch related videos or listen to music together. You could also find websites that offer facts, trivia and other interesting information. Lastly, consider bringing foods that may be associated with the activity or theme.

The next pages contain descriptions of four different Grab & Go Activity Boxes and how each was used. Hopefully they will inspire you to create your special Grab & Go Activity Box.

Al's Baseball Grab & Go Activity Box

Al just loved baseball. He played as a young boy, and later helped coach his son's baseball team. He always watched the Detroit Tigers on television, and attended as many games as he could. Although Al does not remember the names of players on the Tigers team, or even how to keep score, he is still able to reminisce about going to the games.

Al's Box

Al's son Adam put together a Baseball Grab & Go Activity Box to help engage his father. The items were carefully selected based upon Al's love for the game and his favorite team, and included:

- Baseball glove and baseball
- Tigers baseball cap
- Tigers baseball pennant
- Tigers baseball cards
- Box of peanuts
- Small American flag
- Words to the National Anthem
- Words to "Take Me Out to the Ballgame"
- Small book of baseball facts and trivia

How the Box was Used

Al would light up when Adam came in with the box. He loved putting on the Detroit Tigers baseball cap, talking about the team, and looking at the baseball cards that he and his son collected. They had fun singing "Take Me Out to the Ballgame" together. Al derived great pleasure from holding a real baseball and putting on a baseball glove.

To enhance the experience, Adam would sometimes bring hot dogs wrapped up in aluminum foil, along with a 'soda pop' and peanuts. Al remarked that he felt like he was back at the ballpark. On other visits, his son would bring his portable device so they could watch videos of old Tigers games. Adam would also find baseball websites to share some easy and fun baseball trivia, facts and statistics with his father.

Ideas for Your Baseball Grab & Go Activity Box

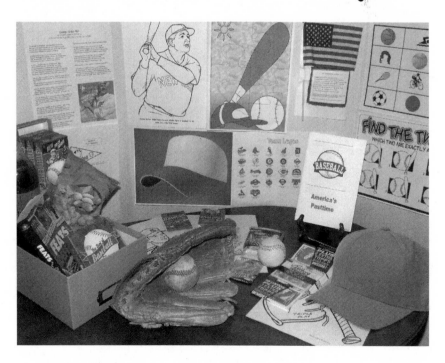

Mary's Bird Grab & Go Activity Box

Mary has always been an avid birder. Her passion started as a young child, when she would sit for hours and watch the birds fly around her backyard. Her two favorite birds were robins and hummingbirds. As an adult, Mary would often take birding vacations and travel to different destinations to see birds in their native habitat.

Mary's Box

Building on Mary's lifelong passion, her daughter Laura put together a Bird Grab & Go Activity Box to help with visits with Mary. This box contained:

- Bird magazines
- Audio book of bird songs
- Small wooden bird house
- Imitation bird nest
- Small packets of different bird seed
- Hummingbird feeder
- Bird calendars
- Picture book of common birds
- Small binoculars
- Adult coloring book with bird pictures
- Song sheet for "When the Red Robin Comes Bobbin Along"

How the Box was Used

Mary loves everything in her box, but her favorite treasure is the Bird Songs book. She got tickled hearing the birds, especially the robin. Mary and her daughter would then sing the "Red Robin" song. Mary also enjoyed looking at bird calendars, and could often name the birds. She would then reminisce about all the different birds she has seen. Laura would also take out the hummingbird feeder and remind her mother that she taught her how to make sugar solution. Mary remembers calling the hummingbirds her "little babies."

When Mary's grandchildren visited, they pulled out some of the bird magazines and made a bird collage together. Another time, they took out the bird house and they decorated it together.

In addition to the Grab & Go Activity Box, Laura would bring her portable device so they could watch bird videos together.

Ideas for Your Bird Grab & Go Activity Box

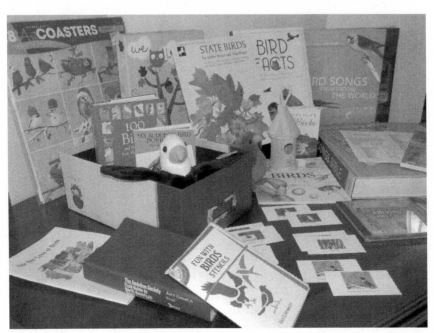

Kathy's Seashore Grab & Go Activity Box

Kathy lived most of her life on the Florida coast near the beach. Her favorite activities revolved around water. Kathy's dementia was such that she had very little short-term memory, but her long-term memory was still intact. The activity box helped her remember those past experiences.

Kathy's Box

Kathy's box was created by her adult children, David and Carol. They knew how much their mother loved the beach, so they put together a seashore themed activity box. Inside they put:

- Sea shells of different shapes, colors and sizes
- A large conch shell
- Sand dollar
- Beach sand
- Blow-up beach ball
- Sun tan lotion
- Pictures of the beach
- Small stuffed dolphin and crab
- Picture book of shells

How the Box was Used - David would take the shells and Kathy would have fun looking at the different colors and textures. He would also talk about how he and his mother used to look for sea shells on the beach. On another visit, Carol pulled out a small stuffed crab and shared memories of walking on the beach at night with flashlights looking for crabs. Knowing how much her mother loved crab cakes, Carol would sometimes bring crab cakes for the two of them to eat together.

When Kathy's eleven-year-old grandson would visit, he would use the small stuffed dolphin to read a dolphin story book. He also brought his smart phone to show his grandmother dolphin videos, which Kathy took much delight in watching. All of these activities brought her much pleasure.

Ideas for Your Seashore Grab & Go Activity Box

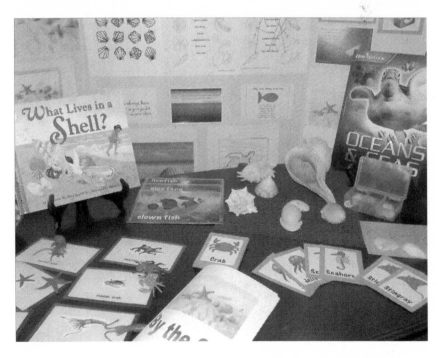

Sam's Tool Grab & Go Activity Box

Sam never really had any hobbies, but did enjoy tinkering with gadgets and fixing things around the house. He also helped fix all sorts of things for his neighbors. Sam has been quite withdrawn and difficult to engage in activities.

Sam's Box

Sam's box was put together by his brother, George. He bought a tool box and filled it with:

- Hammer
- Different size screw drivers
- Pliers
- Level
- Clamp
- Adjustable wrench
- Tape measure
- Bolts and nuts
- Sanding block
- Tool magazines

How the Box was Used - George brought the Tool Grab & Go Activity Box whenever he visited. Sam loved the box and would take out the various items and explain what they were. He particularly loved using the sanding block on an old wooden walking cane. He also had fun adjusting the wrenches and using the clamp. George was able to reminisce with Sam about all the things in the house that he fixed over the years.

Since Sam used to like to tinker with all sorts of things, one day George brought over an old clock. Sam loved taking it apart. George also encouraged Sam's neighbors to bring some different tools and try to engage Sam in reminiscing about fixing things in their homes. The neighbors found a fun way to be with him!

Ideas for Your Tool Grab & Go Activity Box

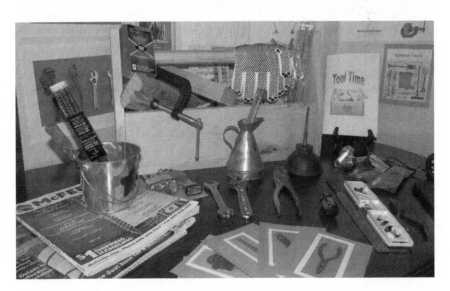

A Grab & Go Box in Use

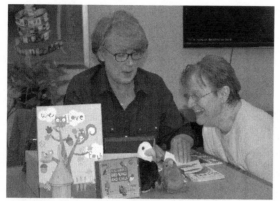

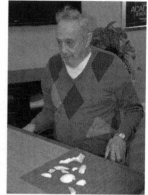

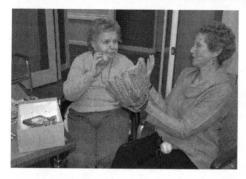

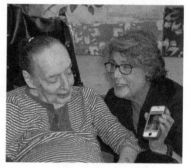

In Summary

Hopefully these ideas will inspire you to create your special Grab & Go Activity Boxes. The boxes can be easy and fun to put together. Care partners have been pleasantly surprised by how receptive their loved ones are to these boxes and how much fun they can have together.

For additional ideas, see

www.meaningfulconnections-dementia.com

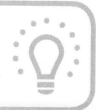

Appendix B

This appendix offers information about creative programs and resources, as well as selected websites for items that can be used for engagement. I hope you will find this information helpful. My clients have appreciated these resources and have found them useful in making positive connections.

Alzheimer's Poetry Project describes the power of using poetry for people with dementia. The site includes videos of how poetry was successfully used to produce 'creative sparks' in people with dementia.

www.alzpoetry.com

Alzheimer's Store provides educational resources and sells health-related products to help make life easier for your loved one with dementia.

www.alzstore.com

Best Alzheimer's Products provides educational information for care partners and also sells a variety of products for those who have dementia.

www.best-alzheimers-products.com

Librivox offers free audio books that are read by volunteers from around world. A variety of topics are available.

www.librivox.org

LifeSongs sells a 12-page scrapbook that a care partner can use to create a "lifesong" with his own voice, along with familiar music, poetry, prayers or stories.

www.lifesongs.info

Lynch Robertson Landscape Architects has a tab on their website dedicated to dementia gardens. Their unique program suggests ways to help those with dementia stay in touch with nature through gardening.

www.dementiasensorygardens.co.uk

Mind Start sells different types of puzzles, activity games, and books designed for those living with dementia.

www.mind-start.com

Music and Memory describes their program in which people with dementia can listen to their favorite music using portable devices and ear phones. The website outlines the profound positive effects on memory, engagement and mood. Care partners can also view video clips from a documentary, "Alive Inside," which uses this approach.

www.musicandmemory.org

Song Writing Works is an organization that promotes the importance of using music in the life of a person with dementia. The website provides videos examples of how music is used.

www.songwritingworks.org

SpringBok sells puzzles specifically developed for people with Alzheimer's disease.

www.springbok-puzzles.com

TimeSlips describes how to use storytelling to engage with a loved one with dementia and offers free storytelling software. Friends and family can create a story by clicking on the "collaborate" button.

www.timeslips.org

Wiser Now Inc., sells a variety of items for those who have dementia, including CDs, printable games, and puzzles.

www.wisernow.com

Updates and additional resources can be found on the book's website:

www.meaningfulconnections-dementia.com

Write Your Notes Here:

61532914R00069

Made in the USA
Lexington, KY
13 March 2017